MW01127281

Why Did God Make Me?

The Spiritual Writings of a
Sparkled-Eyed Man
with Cerebral Palsy

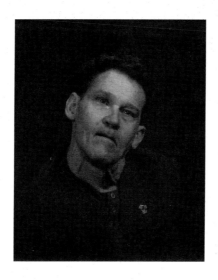

John Raymond "Brother" Groebl

1930-2013

Why Did God Make Me?
Copyright © 2017, John Raymond Groebl

ISBN: 978-1-54392-341-4

A Collection of Poems
And Short Stories

Written by
John "Brother" Groebl

Compiled by
The Loving Family of "Brother"

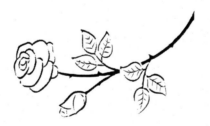

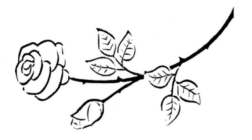

Dedication

This Book is Dedicated to the loving
Parents of Brother

John Peter Groebl

1899–1996

Marie Elizabeth Moeller Groebl

1899–1987

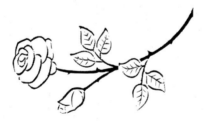

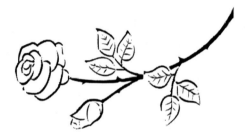

Contents

Introduction

One Finger Speaks My Truth!

By

Sister Louis M. Benecke, SSND

and Oscar J Groebl, Jr.

Simply I write because I like to write. It's not easy as any writer knows, but there's a feeling of accomplishment in the final product.

John "Brother" Groebl

The Poems, Stories, Scripts shared herein, express the goodness beauty, and spaciousness of John's faith filled soul. "Brother", as John was lovingly known by family and friends, believed, accepted, and surrendered to the full reality of being born with severe Cerebral Palsy, CP leaving him dependent upon the care of his parents, family and friends. Yet, despite this he never lost his drive and responsibility of his purpose to speak His Truth of being with love.

To quote John, "Every intelligent person (and thank God He gave me the whole brain) desires a place in the world. Truthfully life is a burden- the burden of love of life and love must express itself in some way."

Physical limitations called forth his creative gifts of gardening and writing. Sometimes crawling on the ground outside "as a worm," his gaze fell on the plants, flowers, trees, and the mystery of their creation and growth from small roots and seeds. Thankfully, John often used a little red wagon to slowly, but steadily inch his way around the garden to care for the simple wonders of nature that defined the universe in a backyard he knew as home. It was here, as well as in front of his typewriter, that John was in control and could freely express his inner and outer love and creativity.

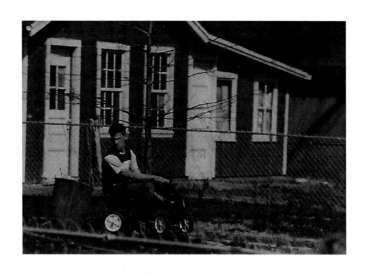

*Brother hard at work in his garden with the
help of his faithful red wagon. 1977*

"Brother" grew into a skilled gardener because, as he wrote, "so much of me must go into everything I do." Gardening graced him to believe in and grow a spaciousness of soul for the Mystery of God. He believed steadfastly that within the small roots and seeds he nurtured, as well as the hearts, minds and souls he touched, plants of all sorts would blossom into flowers.

Needing to share his inner experiences of the mystery of being, John began his efforts to write one letter at a time. Patiently, with courageous "guts" John created a technique that used his left hand to hold his right wrist, guiding one finger to work for him, letter by letter, as he plunked out his words of love and wisdom. One hand led the other, both guided by his internal compass and by the same God who stewarded the seasons coming and going through his wondrous world of the backyard of his physical world.

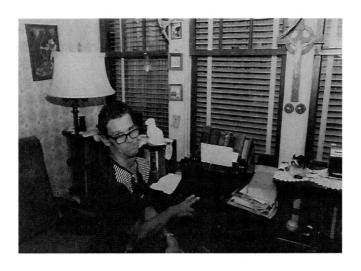

Brother at his desk and typewriter. 1977

Indeed, John has left all of us who love him a legacy of words that reflects his truth mirroring the God who made Him "as fresh as the morning!"

Through this book, we hope that His truth can be shared with those who did not know our "Brother" and help us all to come to know our own strengths and powers and to share our own blossoms with those around us.

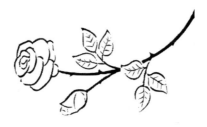

Bringing Together the Author's Words

Are we handicaps being really honest with ourselves by giving the established religious answer to the question, "Would we have wanted to be born had we known we would be handicapped?"

Was I being brainwashed by wrong believers? Was our family doctor right when he told my dad that I wouldn't be happy when I got older? Am I really that miserable?

Yes, I am, but only when I'm barred from doing something that I know I could do with a little guts.

If anything, my books and discussions with people have taught me that WE are the makers of our own prison or our own freedom.

John "Brother" Groebl, 1969

The Spirit Of The Book

Up until the 1960's the fundamental and assumed text for Catholic instruction was based upon a doctrine of forms and teachings called "The Baltimore Catechism". This was the first catechism written for Catholics in North America. It remained in use in nearly all Catholic schools from 1885 until the fresh winds of Vatican II had far reaching and soul touching impact upon every Catholic.

The Baltimore Catechism presented its lessons and teaching through an ongoing list of easily memorized questions. The fourth question, and therefore one of the most important questions was, **"Why did God make you?"**

The answer to this deceptively simple question states, "God made me to know Him, to love Him and to serve Him in this world, and to be happy with Him forever in heaven."

Even though Vatican Council II updated and even did away with many articles of the Baltimore Catechism, aspects of it remain guiding principles for many Catholics. Such was the case for Brother. The challenge of the fourth question, "Why did God Make Me?" always motivated and guided him.

But, to be honest, as we read in the opening quotation, Brother often wrote, even boasted of his spiritual and intellectual radicalism as he struggled with the fourth question. In the small passage below, you will find the extent of his struggles and his posthumous challenges to us.

> *Years ago, if a certain motion picture was condemned I would have been the first one to see it, if I could have gotten to the theater on my own. All these years this same radicalism was bottled up in me!*

Because Brother's faith seemed to have been built soundly upon the Baltimore Catechism His writings are grouped by these three reasons to know Him, to love Him and to serve Him.

However, be ever vigilant for the strong emotional and physical expressions of Brother's ever-present radicalism. For that radicalism is there, tucked among the intentional pauses, exclamation points and needle-sharp questions!

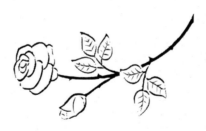

A Bit of Family History

To understand Brother, you need to understand his family, not only his immediate family, but his equally supportive extended family and the generations of strong German traditions that were the foundations of the family's day to day existence.

St. Louis was heavily populated in the 1840's and then again in the 1880's by Germans seeking new opportunities and freedoms away from the "old country". Brother's great grandparents were among those fleeing emigrants and as such, they instilled in all subsequent generations focus, fight and a striving for success. Brother himself wrote of life, *"persistence, reinforced by courage!"*

One of John's poems calls back from the past the love, the structure, the community and even the smell of "Papa's nightly bucket of beer."

The family eventually moved away from the close quarters above the Butcher Shop and into a home, all their own and one with a backyard that evolved into Brother's haven of gardening, contemplation and the ever-loving nurturing of God's iris', roses, daffodils, and the peonies.

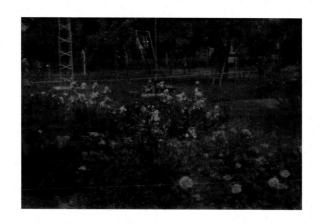

Brother's backyard world, the magical place where God's love, John's courage, persistence and knowledge, and the pollinating bees of nature all came together.

Thus, It Was Back Then

Published in New Voices In American Poetry 1980

"Fetch down the chair, Papa."

Mamma would call though the hall,

Even though Papa would be coming down the stairs

with the wooden folding chair,

Now the stairs and hall are still there;

so are the rooms upstairs where Mamma and Papa

Below still is the store

then called "The Butcher Shop",

When Mamma and Papa sat out in front there on

summer evenings,

trying to catch a breath of the warm scented air.

Each store, for there were many back then;

the row broken only by yards and hallways

that were never feared,

gave off a certain scented breath

that told of their wares inside,

which were mixed with the street fumes outside,

but back then it meant more life than death.

A jeweler had the corner back then

and stayed open sometimes 'til almost ten,

cleaning clocks and watches with an

intermittent spray

heard through door left opened wide.

The pendulum clock on the window side wall would

strike nine,

and folks would stir from their stoops and benches.

Wagons and tricycles were put away.

'til the morrow, when they would once again throttle

over make -believe trenches.

Alas.

But now it was time for Papa's nightly bucket of beer

while Mamma went down for her orange pop,

which she didn't think would harm her diabetes any,

Mamma went real fast—

down in the country one weekend.

Papa was real lonesome then,

and pretty soon joined Mamma at eternal rest

Thus, is was back then.

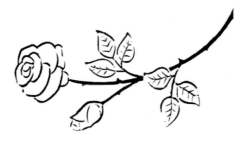

In the Author's Own Words

My face might seem like an expressionless mask.

Though I speak

*Somehow the words don't seem to do
justice to my heart's task —*

Just to be understood; not necessarily to reform,

That's all I ask.

From *My Heart's Task*

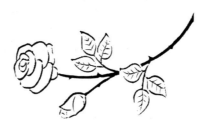

Real Barriers To Overcome

There are certain things that really bug us handicaps besides physical barriers, which generally can be overcome with self-determination and a good sense of humor. However, the emotional barriers that we either create for ourselves or that Mr. Right creates for us are what sometimes make us home handicaps shut-ins, if not totally physical than mental. My story mainly concerns itself with these home handicaps since I'm one of them. The emotional barriers are created around what I call the five categories of living. Ironically, Mr. Right also inhibits himself somewhat by imposing these barriers on us.

The first of these categories I've entitle "Friends and Lovers". It seems that Mr. Right has a tendency to put all handicapped persons into one big collection basket, as he does with all minorities. In mixed company, for example, the nineteen-year-old paraplegic is supposed to make friends with the forty-five-year-old cerebral palsied person and the eighty-year-old stroke victim is supposed to become friends with both. Believe it or not, my own sister once even put a person with "a denture" into that basket.

Now perhaps they will all hit it off together, not because of any common physical abilities or disabilities, but because of that natural certain something that attracts friends, although it would be perhaps psychologically unrealistic to say that the former didn't have a little something to do with it. On the other hand, two cerebral palsied persons might not be able to tolerate each other.

Oh yes, we have prejudice among us too; perhaps even a more severe kind. If we have any hang-ups at all about ourselves seeing another person in almost the same physical condition is surely like looking into a mirror; we have our good, bad, and those in between. For diversion then we like to make friends with normal people our own age, who aren't so apt to patronize us and who are still abled bodied enough to take us places. And we might even teach each other a thing or two.

My next category appropriately is "Sex". I daresay that most of us presently middle-aged home handicaps had to learn about sex on our own. The dictionary was one of my main sources of information. Not only because parents didn't discuss such things in those days, but in our parents', eyes we were still seven and eight years old during our adolescence. I've always felt that because of my physical disabilities I was about ten to fifteen years behind mentally. Our parents were certain that we would never marry. So, what would have been the purpose in dirtying our innocent little minds with sex? And subconsciously they finally had a way, through us, to keep a child in the cradle of purity – some psychological parental hang-up in human nature.

However, nature wouldn't submit to this silence. In fact, because of it she seemed to be screaming even louder. Surprisingly, some of us were able to go out and silence her, if only for a short time. Those of us who haven't found a way out yet duplicate her screams for sex like a starving man screams for food.

Not to sound sacrilegious but just honest, at times I strive not for the perfect happiness of the next world, as I was taught to endeavor for, but for a perfect sexual union with someone of this world. At times I make sex my ultimate goal in life while at the same time I fool Mr. Right into believing that I have a monk's fortitude.

And yet through all of this, I can be pretty snobbish and particular about sex. I find physically abnormal females somewhat sexually unattractive. I hunger after the blossoming normal girls.

After that, I'd better go on to my third category "Religion". No one in my circle of physically handicapped friends feel that he or she has any special link with God because of their disabilities. One is a nonbeliever while the others are of mixed faiths. I guess that I was once too halfway talked into believing something like this as I once believed that I had some special link with Him just because I was Catholic. But some reading and Pope John XXIII seemed to have helped stop these ego trips.

Personally, I've become a firm believer in the reincarnation theory – the only reasonable explanation for all the unequaled illness in the world. Somewhat shockingly at first after all the sentimentality, it told me that my soul chose to come back in this present cerebral palsied body in repentance for sins committed in former life.

In order to read and think, we had to have some sort of elementary education, which brings us to my fourth category. But neither is our intelligence taken for granted. Because Mr. Right sees so little of what we home handicaps can actually do at our own IQ level and physical pace and because for the most part our outward expressions generally don't make us appear too intelligent, especially if our handicap is from brain damage, he overreacts with our display of intelligence before him. This in turn, if the reaction is favorable, can give us a wrong sense of accomplishment and lead us into believing something about ourselves that isn't necessarily true, especially if we're the least bit praise and attention hungry. He might be so impressed by my being able to write a simple letter that he gives me the impression that I can become a novelist.

On the other hand, if his reaction is unfavorable to our sensibility, we might accuse him of thinking us mentally retarded, and we might exclaim: "I'll show him." Well, as time passes he generally forgets what he said, and we spend our energy proving something to a ghost. So, when it comes to education, we should realize that we also have our genuine PhDs, High School dropouts, and those in between.

Because Mr. Right usually tries so hard to protect us, it can be somewhat of an affront to him for us to say that we also have our fears, which brings us to my fifth and last category.

I can see why it might be hard for him, who might see us all crippled up in wheelchairs, to realize that we too fear old age, illness, and death. Perhaps we fear the first two a trifle more because (I'm thinking mainly of us palsied persons) our muscular movements aren't isolated. For example, I couldn't type last summer because of a sprained big toe. My toes even move when I talk. And like Mr. Right we're concerned just how we're going to die; we don't have any special guardian angel telling us what's on the other side.

Those persons who are able to go out working on crutches and in wheelchairs are also concerned about losing their jobs. Again, even more so because they just can't walk or roll into any kind of job.

I think one of the biggest concerns for us middle-aged home handicaps requiring custodial care such as having to be helped get dressed, fed, etc. is what's going to happen to us when our parents pass away and there's no immediate family to care for us. Since this could happen at any time, we're concerned that we'll have to spend the rest of our young days in some old folks' home, awaiting death when we still have so many plans for ourselves.

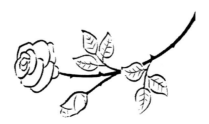

Learning to Know

When we speak to a true friend
We do not speak from a prepared text;
We say what is in our heart.
We speak from the depths of our soul.
Now, we can speak to God this way,
His presence is all around us.
For instance, do you speak to your plants?
No, I do not jest,
because to behold such love for anything,
and utterance from the lips
which starts from the soul must come - from a prayer.

From a Draft of *What is Prayer?*

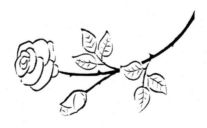

The World Still Awaits

There's that time of day

when I must quietly be alone

to reflect; to meditate; to pray;

call it what you will.

Present are my God and those in spirit near and far;

even those beyond the stars.

Now this may be selfishness enhanced,

for His real world still awaits

with its love, laughter and ills;

not to be shut out and left alone

but to be changed.

Nothing But Still A Lot

O dear Lord,

Please tell me

Who am I?

What am I?

Where am I?

Where have I been?

Where am I going?

He says:

No body.

Nothing.

No where.

No where.

And I cry out

in despair.

Please repair.

Prayer
To Those Who Feel Joy

What is prayer?

A morning touched by the emerald dew

or even a freshly fallen snow

and my being swells with exaltation,

bringing to my lips words of joy and appreciation

For this day anew,

This to me is one form of prayer.

The Poet At Lent

What do I see on Easter morn?

I see a freshened earth after a storm.

An earth bursting forth in all its glory,

An earth that is calm again after its fury.

I see a white robed figure treading the land.

He wears a beard and walks with staff in hand,

While a pure white dove shepherds on high.

I must speak to Him before He passes me by.

But what did I see on a day before that

glorious morn?

I saw an earth grow dark before the storm,

An earth that would trembled under angry skies,

An earth that would blow dust into my eyes.

I saw a tattered robed figure treading a path.

I have often traveled myself this rocky path.

He wore a beard and shouldered a cross.

And I have many times felt the weight of that cross.

Happy Birthday

As nature's other things of spring

we children of March, April and May

seem to have a something all our own

as a potential bursting

that sometimes stretches the sinew beyond

    endurance

and make us seem to lack tolerance,

but then comes the bloom without delay

and nothing could be more fulfilling.

        To Aunt Mary March 1984

        Dorothy March 1984

        Aunt Bert April 1984

Tints Of Gold

What is as refreshing as a summer's evening

    after a shower?

The clouds part to let the sun have its

    final hour.

And the world becomes tinted with orange

    and gold,

'il the morning smog once again takes hold.

Just One Seed And Many Trees

I planted a seed

from which after much care and nurturing

a seedling grew

which gradually became a fruit bearing tree.

Now, some of its fruit ripened ever so sweetly

while others were sour tasting

and still others shriveled and browned

but clung desperately to the swaying branches

as the winds grew raw.

While still other dropped to the ground in

injured dismay;

their skins rotting away,

and their seeds laying bare to the rains and snows,

But Mother Nature was kind in her usual way

and blanketing them with her soil

until it was time for the earth to be renewed

and lo and behold many trees grow.

A Summer's Evening Symphony

Published in New Voices American Poetry 1979

O dear robin red breast

from greenery to greenery

from street treetop,

where locusts also sing,

to backyard grapevine

you keep an open line,

chirping back and forth in sweet evening song.

The message is yours alone

Your notes, however, seem to come from the rainbow

across the eastern sky-

bars of reds, oranges, and blues

and the gold in the West

(a few hours ago a raging Luzon)

now completes the symphony at its best,

playing the twilight overture.

Then quieter and quieter the music

as the conductor gently lowers his golden baton,

and the velvet curtain studded with a thousand

twinkling stars descends.

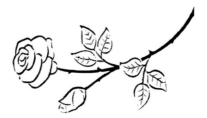

Falling Leaves

Why do we sometimes look upon the falling

    leaves as drops of tears

When they could be our troubles scattering?

Why do we say the autumn of our years

When there must be an autumn for a spring?

Why must we curse the frozen earth

When it's the frost that helps the seed

    make a tree?

Spring too you see brings death as well as birth.

The Trash Truck Cometh

With a crunch, whine, and grind

through the ice and snow

The trash man cometh.

Now hurry,

gone with

you symbols of that holy night surprise;

beckoning; tempting to hands and eyes.

Held gently and all aglow

With the rest of the decked-out warmth.

Then perhaps laid aside.

Now suddenly dumped and crushed

and rushed out into the cold and snow.

You're a soreness to the eye.

My Flying Friends

O my dear flying friends,

Perched high atop that watchtower,

chirping your little hearts out.

Listen! And laugh a little too.

I don't blame you because here comes what is

       supposed to be an imitation of you.

And with one supersonic boom

we're both off in the blue.

But let me ask you this

while we're up here above the storm.

Were your bags packed

And your bank account stacked

And your motors gassed and oiled?

How long did you have to "please stand-by"/

And are your seat belts strapped?

Therefore, my flying friends,

Without a doubt, you are still the true masters

       of the skies.

The Rains Came

The rains came and washed gullies in the soil

Like tears wash into the soul.

The sun comes out and dries the land,

But the ruts still remain.

Even growth begins.

Tears are dried by the hand,

But only time's warmth can heal the soul,

And too growth begins.

Snow Mounds

Mounds of snow piled against curb and gutter,

Once pure and white in angelical flutter;

individualism behold,

But then pushed and shoved in lumps dirty and sooty

to clear the streets for man's city.

Tommy, God's Plan...

With our hospitals and other institutions so crowded even the holiest of us might wonder why God permits this suffering and at times even ask: Where is He? Well, far be it for me to know the answer. However, each time I receive Holy Communion or now laugh it up with the members of HEC I can't help thinking back to a day in July 1948 when a young parish priest, who I shall call Father K and who has since passed away, came up to see my two-week-old nephew Tommy. I was eighteen at the time and since I was attending public school I wasn't receiving any sort of religious instructions and starting to be concerned about my salvation. What if I should suddenly die...? Anyway, to make a long story short, Mom mentioned this to Father K as she did to so many other priests previously. However, this time the phone rang the following Easter Monday evening. and it was Father K. I'd like to come up and see John, he said which started tens weeks of religious instructions after school each Monday and which ended with a private first Holy Communion Mass in the sacristy of the Church of the Epiphany.; As for Tommy, He's a man living at the St. Louis School and Hospital for the severely retarded. Was that day in July 1948 just a coincidence because by now I would have probably made my Communion somehow or was it Tommy's fulfillment in life- somehow all in God's plan? Since I am a romantic, like to think the latter, but I'll leave the real answer up to the scholars. Anyway, thanks Tommy, certainly not for your retardation but for accepting God's Plan.

Learning to Know

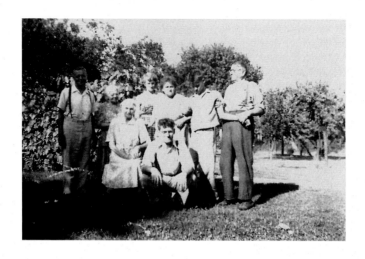

Brother's family was a critical factor of his loving and supportive life. Brother's parents, grandparents, sister and extended family provided unlimited and unconditional love. They knew God's gifts in his special needs and talents.

Pictured here:

Front row, kneeling: John Peter Groebl, Father

Second row, sitting in chair: Grandmother Anna Schaan Groebl

Back Row: Grandfather Oscar J. Groebl, Sr.; Catherine Moeller, Aunt; Dorothy Groebl Rothery, Sister; Brother himself; Marie Moeller Groebl, Mother; and Grandfather Michael B. Moeller

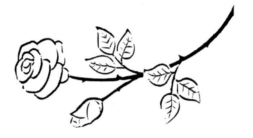

Learning to Love

Truthfully it is a burden; the burden
of love of life and of love.

Love must express itself in many ways.

John "Brother" Groebl, 1969

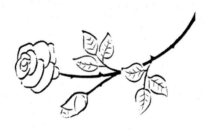

God's Grace

What will grant me for today?

Will it be darkened skies

Or bright sunlight?

If I'm in His grace,

I don't fear the darkest skies,

but if I'm out of His grace no matter how much

I fear the brightest sunlight.

The Game Of Twenty-One

When I was a mere boy of ten and one,

I couldn't wait 'til I was a man of twenty-one.

When I was a mere man of twenty-one,

I couldn't wait 'til I was a giant at fifty-one.

After I was a mere giant at fifty-one.

I thought that I was God at eighty-one.

Perhaps when I'm a hundred and one (God willing)

I'll be that unique one.

Or will I still be looking for that magical one.

A Tribute To The First Flowers
Of Spring

Come now all you first flowers of spring;

don't let this chilly April morning get you down.

Lift up those drooping heads and wear that crown,

for you represent a rebirth.

You are the little princesses of the universe

touched by some magic wand.

Look Beyond The Clouds

Thus, damp and gloomy grow the days,

and my thoughts turn to those in eternal slumber.

Soaked in puddles of heavenly rains leaves lay

as my heart is in human tears.

The world seems cast in a darkened shroud

And yet I must put this state of gloom asunder

and look beyond the clouds,

For there still shines that celestial star.

Credit Where Credit's Due

There are hundreds of roses in my yard,

each a different size and color.

Even from the same root it seems

that no two are exactly the same.

Some stand so straight and tall

and hold their own against wind and rain

while others, the slightest breeze makes them fail.

But weak or strong; light or dark, none can I

      disregard

As a mother cannot abandon one child for another,

And as she glories in her triumph after childbirth

so do I also marvel at the beauty that I helped my

      roses bring forth.

Their roots and stalks were not developed by me,

      however,

this was done by someone much smarter than I,

And it's the root that makes the plant and flower;

So what good would it do me to complain about

      their form,

For it's a little late now to return the plants;

I got what I'd ordered, and all roses have thorns.

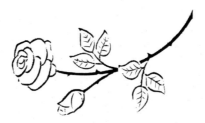

So Many Memories

So many memories I have stored;

So demanding to be heard.

But how to find the words.

So selfishly I keep silent, remembering

    and dreaming

and not sharing those recollections

and those memories that should make our

    life together.

And yet every man has a right to life's

    silent reflections.

The Reason Why

The skies are leaden with clouds of gray;

There's a scent of snow in the air.

But that feeling of warmth lies within me.

As I rake the last of fall's remains away.

It seems odd to be raking in this yuletide atmosphere,

For no rustling leaves or robin's songs stir the sir.

Mother Nature's earth seems to be dead,

Distance church chimes I hear instead.

Discordantly the first noel sounds over the

leadened air.

The East wind stirs and excites something within me.

I sense decked out downtown in its colorful array.

But to travel still farther East would thrill me

even more

and to be in the little town of Bethlehem would really

stir me.

And see the reason why I felt this way today.

But farther East my imagination travels to a

small town

where the baby Jesus lay,

and that's why I feel this way today.

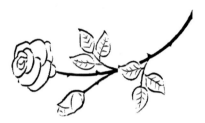

The Oak Tree, My Love

See the giant oak tree, my love,

Reaching toward the heavens above

Beneath, its roots so firm and deep in Mother earth;

also reaching and competing for nourishment

from the ground around,

making its branches and leaves so sound,

sheltering God's tiny creatures from night storms.

And yet the sun filters through,

giving strength to other births.

The Thanksgiving Day Scene

Steam on windowpanes

Smells in the air

From food on the stove a cookin'

Hands a reachin' and a grabbin'

Tableware a clankin'

Voices a soundin'

But none a speakin'

Then a tinkin'

And silence

And prayer.

Quiet Reflections

So many memories I have stored;

so demanding to be heard.

And now with a beloved by my side

even more so with pride.

But how to find the words

is the affliction.

so selfishly to myself I keep

these events passed,

remembering and dreaming even before I sleep.

but they are the past!

And yet every man has a right to those quiet

reflections.

Eternal Bliss

There shines in the heaven eternal

three stars looking down on this sixtieth nuptial,

awaiting in joyous gladness for Mom and Dad.

While two other children standing holding perhaps

not physically even so tightly the love shared.

remembering the happy times along with the sad;

the laughter and the tears.

The children reach out for the weakened body

and the bewildered mind.

The son knows that the parting of the ways is

    but temporary,

for there in the heavens four more will shine

    in eternal bless.

"To My Dad"

I see him in twilight,

laying his weary body upon sheets of white.

I see him in the morning,

struggling to get his weary body out of bed.

I see him at noon,

coming through the gate

so straight and tall,

pulling his shopping cart

filled with food for all----

      All?

Now there's just the two of us

where there used to be eight of us.

Then suddenly one morning

he had a fall:

bruised and broken

he didn't say anything at all

until one morning

while making his usual Friday pancakes

he finally complained that his arm still ached.

so to the doctor he went,

but still so straight and tall.

Now that was not the end of the story,

for he lived for four more years;

so why should I shed tears

When I know that he's in his heavenly glory.

Just Who Was She?

Published in American Poetry 1979

A dear, sweet mamma in rocking chair and shawl,

I'm certain that you don't recall.

it was on Saturdays

while you were busy helping Daddy in the store,

and we kids. Dorothy and I, had to go up to

    Grandma's.

I guess that we always used "up" because grandma

    lived on the second floor

and the street, Gravois, ran "up" from us.

Behind Grandma's was a potato chip factory

with pungent odors and 5am shifts.

Anyway, it was there that I remember this old lady—

Well, she mightn't have been all that old.

It was just how she looked in red scarf, thin

    black coat,

which she wore even on warm days, and tennis shoes,

and what she did that made her look quite used, and

    us amused.

She looked the part of distrust.

And I was only about six or seven at the time.

I remember playing out on the back porch floor

and peering down through the wooden slats

when down the alley she came with bag and parcel,

picking from each can from which rodents ran any

     potato morsel

not fit to be fried, packed and sold.

Now either she was a madam of thrift

or a victim of the times,

for it during what I later learned were the Great

     Depression Days,

Now I think of them as the good times

even though there were some scary times.

I am now in my late forties and remembering

but why am I asking

as I embrace you in rocking chair and shawl

and Grandma's picture on the wall.

Just who was the old lady in red scarf, black thin coat

     and tennis shoes?

"If You Should Remember Me"

When I am in my grave so cold and little,

Remember me, I say;

But weep little,

For rather would I have you remember and be happy

and gay.

But when I am gone away,

I do say this, weep you shall,

If you have harmed me in any way.

For a moment or two you may bow your head

and dwell.

But then I implore you again be merry and gay.

For me do not sob or pout,

When I am gone forever away,

For I am happy, tis without a doubt.

Enjoy life as I once did,

Before I took that last trip,

And they closed the lid.

Pray that I took the right ship.

Again, I tell you, remember me when I am gone away,

But weep small or not at all;

Rather would I have you pray,

For now, in my grave I am quite helpless and small.

When I am gone to my last appointment to keep,

Just remember, pray but smile,

Pray not only for my soul to keep,

But for those who must still travel that last

treacherous mile.

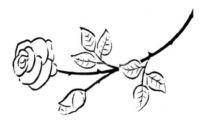

Learning to Love

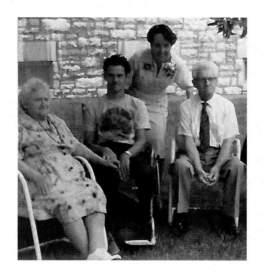

In addition to Brother's immediate family, his extended
family provided the love and support to go beyond his
physical challenges. Aunts, Uncles, cousins were there for
him with unconditional acceptance; nurturing Brother,
just as he nurtured the plants in his garden.

Pictured here:

Left to Right: Marie Moeller Groebl, Mother; Brother himself;
Sr. Louise Benecke, SSND, Cousin; John Peter Groebl, Father

The occasion was the 25th Jubilee of Sr. Louise's
commitment to the School Sisters of Notre Dame at
the order's Mother house in St. Louis, Missouri

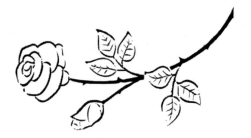

Learning to Serve

*We have the power to take our life between our hands
and mold it into a bright view we can gaze upon.*

Seeking! Searching! Finding!

John "Brother" Groebl, 1969

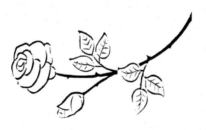

A Writer's Lament

Alone, at the typewriter I sit moodily

 a genius at work, supposedly,

Trying to set words to rhyme

 and down thoughts that are mine,

While out there the true drama unfolds,

 for the world is not a stage, I'm told,

with us as performers making daily debuts.

Now, please permit one more to enter from the wings

and write the epitaphs and reviews

about the sad faces and the clowns

about their ups and their downs.

Perhaps he can give some correct "on cues"

then he will exit, too,

and the chorus shall sing

as another sad faced clown passes in review.

Faith In The Crown Of Thorns

My mind is a whirlwind of activity.

A torrent of thoughts both simple and of the

difficult variety.

Hush! I so want to command;

look to him with pierced feet and nailed hands;

bow they unsettled soul before hung head and crown

of thorns;

Then arise to that joyous morn.

Yet till thy fields,

But behold the lilies of those fields.

The Strands Of Life

The strands of life stretch and pull

at times.

First this way, then the other

and just when we're about to cry "O Brother"

out comes the sun

and warms and softens them

bringing back in time

until we are ready for another, whatever.

My Heart's Task

My face might seem like an expressionless mask.

Though I speak

Somehow the words don't seem to do justice to my

heart's task -

just to be understood; not necessarily to reform,

that's all I ask.

So strong is the desire within

that some venting must be found.

Perhaps rage; then tears abound,

But then immaturity speaks, and all seem to be

swept away

by the outgoing tide,

And once again I go inside myself and hide.

But then I still have a task to perform -

to satisfy my heart's desire;

Not with rage or tears sired

but with words that are sound.

Glass Houses
To Those In The Public's Eye

A young man in the prime of life

stands proudly beside his wife.

Heroes proclaimed.

Then suddenly the flags become half mast

while she stands black veiled beside a grave.

Now it is asked:

"Were they all that innocent and brave

or was it only a public mask -----

a claim to fame?"

Whichever, this I say:

Whoever made them the other,

Let them take off their mask.

They Make Guns

The make guns to go to war with,

guns to fight crime with,

and guns to hunt animals with.

They even make guns to play with.

But they made one gun too many

when they made the one

that killed my son.

He wasn't an enemy,

A criminal,

Or an animal.

He was only my son.....

My Imprisoned Self

I chained myself to a prison cell;

no judge could have placed me in such a hell.

It was I alone who placed me there,

and it will be I alone who gets me out of there

    alone....

Then why do I pray night and day

for someone to show me the way?

Unseen And Unfulfilled

Open the door to my soul,

and there

you'll find many things

that I so crave:

family, and friends now hopefully at peace,

but still the beauty and challenge of living;

so many things unseen and undone

unfulfilled;

only to rot in my grave

if I allow them to do so.

My Haunted Wish

If I could have but one wish granted,

it would be to turn back the hands of time.

"So granted,"

Says the ever-searching soul within me.

but still it aches and yearns

for the still more tender years

When I was building sand castles in space.

But why am I so attached to this time past,

too taunted

When grown is my wish, haunted.

The Seed Of Growth

Honorable Mention in

"It's A Great Life Poetry Contest" 1987

As a rose must be nourished by the soil's nutrients

so the mind must be nourished by life continuities.

Therefore, be not too glad when a task is fulfilled,

for then boredom and desolation await.

Even death!

No, I say;

look to the next with anticipation.

And life!

For as sure as the universe rotates

It shall come.

Fear not failure

If so hampered,

for it too can be a seed of growth.

St Louis Is Its Name

As I traveled the fifty states and seven continents too,

there burned within me as I went from place to place

a torch for the city of my birth.

I don't' go into detail about my experiences away

from home,

because they were had, I'm quite sure, by many many

times before.

In fact, my lyrics might sound like just numerations,

but I hope not

because each experience whether it be at a crowded

game or alone in some cathedral to reflect

gave me a sense of belonging to a city, a state, a

nation, God's universe- His human race.

I don't even go into detail about the place I sing about

because like every other city it has its good; its bad;'

its old;' its new..

But unlike any other place on earth

It's the city of my birth

and St louis is its name.

Yes, I sailed beneath the Golden Gate

and marveled at the view from atop the Empire State

I watched play in the astrodome

and explored Alaska's frigid zone.

I scorched my feet on desert sands

And crossed rocky badlands.

I visited out of town parks and monuments

And walked through corn country beneath a

harvest moon.

I stood before buildings of parliaments.

and thought of my forefathers looking toward these

distant shores.

I was awed by the holiness of Rome

and grandeur of India's Taj Mahal.

I marveled at the rebirth of Japan

and wade through rice paddies of Vietnam

before reaching a mightier stream

Here, I said a prayer in thanksgiving for its city of

New Orleans.

Now I knew that I would be home soon,

for I passed locks, dams, and barges along the way.

I stepped onto a cobble shore

and above a silvery arch gleamed,

perhaps not yet of world fame,

but this was St. Louis-

the city of my birth.

A Prayer For Success

O Lord, help me to succeed-

Help me reach my goals,

But help me also to take my success in a humble way.

Never let me become too big to remember my

humble beginning,

nor too important to recall those I once knew,

nor too strong to take the weakest hand in mine,

nor too wise to listen to the most confused and

bewildered mind,

nor think myself too pure to help the poor soul who

went astray,

nor let me forget I also could have gone that way,

nor let me become too rich to know the poor

still exist,

nor too independent to know I still need my

fellow man,

nor too busy to lend my neighbor a helping hand,

nor think myself to infallible to be proven wrong,

nor too indispensable to be replaced,

nor too proud to think that mine is the only religion

and the only race,

and finally, and most important of all,

never let me become too powerful to forget Thee.

Yes, O Lord, help me to succeed

but also make that success a proud and happy one.

"About Readin..."

If books are the greatest thing,

then why,

as I learned to read

and my intelligence evolved

has famine, religion and prejudice

become involved?

All unknown before I began.

I Pray That They'll Never Know

Published in New Voices American Poetry 1980

On this bright memorial morning

the world seems without mourning,

for those white crosses all in a row

and their dead sleeping below,

while tiny hands in uniform so neat

so quickly places a tiny flag by each.

unknown why those sleep below

save read in books, perhaps.

The truth, perhaps, and yet not,

for words can never describe

the pain of dying in frozen snow

or thirsting in desert heat.

Lips parched and praying to be reached,

if only by God;

then let it be so.

But I pray that they'll never know.

Learning to Serve

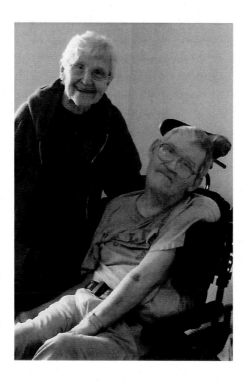

Brother's sister Dorothy Groebl Rothery and her entire family of children and grandchildren were there to serve Brother, helping to fulfill his needs.

Pictured here is Dorothy on a visit to Brother in his care facility toward the end of his life. Dorothy always brought Brother's favorite coffee and ice cream on each visit.

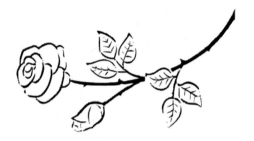

A New Beginning

Why do we sometimes look upon the falling
Leaves as drops of tears
When they could be our troubles scattering?
Why do we say the autumn of our years
When there must be an autumn for a spring?
Why must we curse the frozen earth
When it's the frost that helps the seed
make a tree?
Spring too you see brings death as well as birth.

From *Falling Leaves*

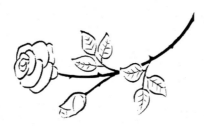

There is never a good day in any month to die; be it on a cold day in the months of winter, a sunny brisk day of spring, a hot and humid day of summer, or an orange, dry day of autumn.

But, for a gardener and lover of nature like Brother, a day in March may be the best possible day, since it is just between the promising days as winter wanes and the teasingly sunny days of spring, each day warming the soil for the seeds yet to be planted in it.

Brother never got to plant any more seeds. John Raymond "Brother" Groebl died on March 30, 2013.

It was a quiet and peaceful death, one befitting a man who wrote of love, of patience, of perseverance and of the cycles of nature.

We will never know what thoughts occupied his mind, what fears, dreams and hopes filled his soul, as his tortured and racked body finally succumbed to the effect of his own variety of Cerebral Palsy.

We hope he was at peace, something well-deserved in exchange for the comfort, strength and inspiration he gave so many others.

Brother was laid to rest in a simple casket; he was dressed in overalls and accompanied by his well-used hand gardening tools. He is buried within the family plot surrounded by his long-deceased grandparents, parents, infant brothers, aunts, uncles and cousins. As in life, he is surrounded in death by loved ones.

Brother has finally overcome his barriers and rests in quiet peace waiting for the day of his resurrection, a resurrection that he so firmly believed in.

However, Brother's own resurrection has already begun through this book of his poems and stories. Even though his body still waits to rise again, his spirit and words live on; inspiring, teaching, and guiding. Each word, shares with the living, you and me, his journey through life to know Him, to love Him and to serve Him.

Each of Brother's words is now planted in us; it is up to us to nourish them, answering for ourselves, "Why Did God Make Me?"

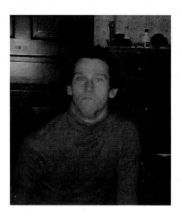

The Tree Bough

O Lord, so many times I want to put my faith and

trust in You.

But then like a tree caught in a breeze

I find myself trembling and shaking and not leaving it

up to You.

O know I should if I only could, but it seems that I

must bend the tree bough my way.

I should know that this is ever so hard to do:

I am only caught up in the sway.

And until You decide to ease the breeze

All that I can do is pray.

Where will it stop, if ever, is all up to You.

All that I can do is hang on and pray.

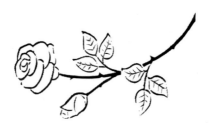

About the Family Contributors

The fifteenth question of the Baltimore Catechism is, "**Where is God?**" The answer is, "God is everywhere."

Brother's writings clearly show that God is indeed everywhere, that His love and support is always available to everyone, but especially to those like Brother who are open to all that He offers.

Over the years Brother's acceptance of his limitation and condition and his embracing the love and support from God inspired many family members. His courage and perseverance inspired close family and friends.

Five family members realized that Brother's journey of life was a light that should be put on a stand to give light to everyone.

In an effort to let Brother's light "shine before all men," these five members, after reading and reflecting on all Brother's writings, compiled, edited and packaged this collection of poetry and writings. May this publication continue Brother's desire to show that God is indeed everywhere, that His Love and support is always available to everyone, but especially to those like Brother who are open to all that He offers.

Dorothy Groebl Rothery

After the death of his parents, Brother's primary caregiver and guardian was his sister, Dorothy Groebl Rothery. Dorothy also lovingly kept the poems and writings presented here and made them available to be shared. Just as God's love was the light in Brother's world, his sister Dorothy and her children were the rock to which Brother would always anchor himself.

Sr. Louise Benecke SSND

Sr. Louise is a 2nd cousin to Brother John through paternal grand- mothers, Anna and Caroline Schaan sisters. As a growing child she became friends with Brother at the Groebl Family gatherings and celebrations. As a religious, mission ministry in the States and overseas deepened the relationship and created a lifelong journey of shared letters, writings, prayer to support Brother's hopes, and dreams. When ministering in Arizona, Sister hosted Brother and Dorothy so they could experience the beauty of God's creation in the Grand Canyon and mountains of Arizona.

Oscar J. Groebl, Jr. (Sonny)

Sonny the son of Oscar J. Groebl, who is a first cousin to Brother. Sonny. the family genealogist, has an awareness of family relationships and his gift of enjoying and gathering the relatives, is the glue that bonded the family team contributors together. His knowledge of the Groebl family background provided the team with appropriate historical sequencing and gave meaningful strands for the placement of the poems and short stories. He also provided the needed transportation to Dorothy and Sister Louise when neither one of them could drive. He had lived in California for many years and was close to Mark and Mary Ann Hutcherson and Mary Ann's mother Bertha Groebl McSwain, the sister of Brother's father, John. When Mark and Mary Ann retired to St. Louis in 2015 Sonny connected all of us together.

Mark and Mary Ann Hutcherson

Upon their return in 2015 Mary Ann and Mark reconnected with the all the family known and unknown. Mary Ann is the youngest of Brother's ten first cousins. They are active members of their parish, Immaculate Conception Dardenne Prairie and volunteer their creative services to the Pauline Books and Media Book Center and the Daughters of St. Paul Community.

After several gatherings these family members began to focus on the possibility of publishing Brother's writings. Each of the members brought complimentary gifts that could place Brother's writings on the lampstand for all to see.

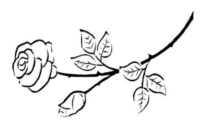

You are the light of the world. A town built on a hill cannot be hidden. Neither do people light a lamp and put it under a bowl. Instead they put it on its stand, and it gives light to everyone in the house. In the same way, let your light shine before all men, that they may see your good deeds and glorify your Father in heaven.

Matthew 5:14-16